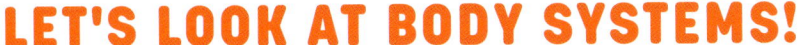

LET'S LOOK AT BODY SYSTEMS!

NOAH'S NIFTY NERVOUS SYSTEM

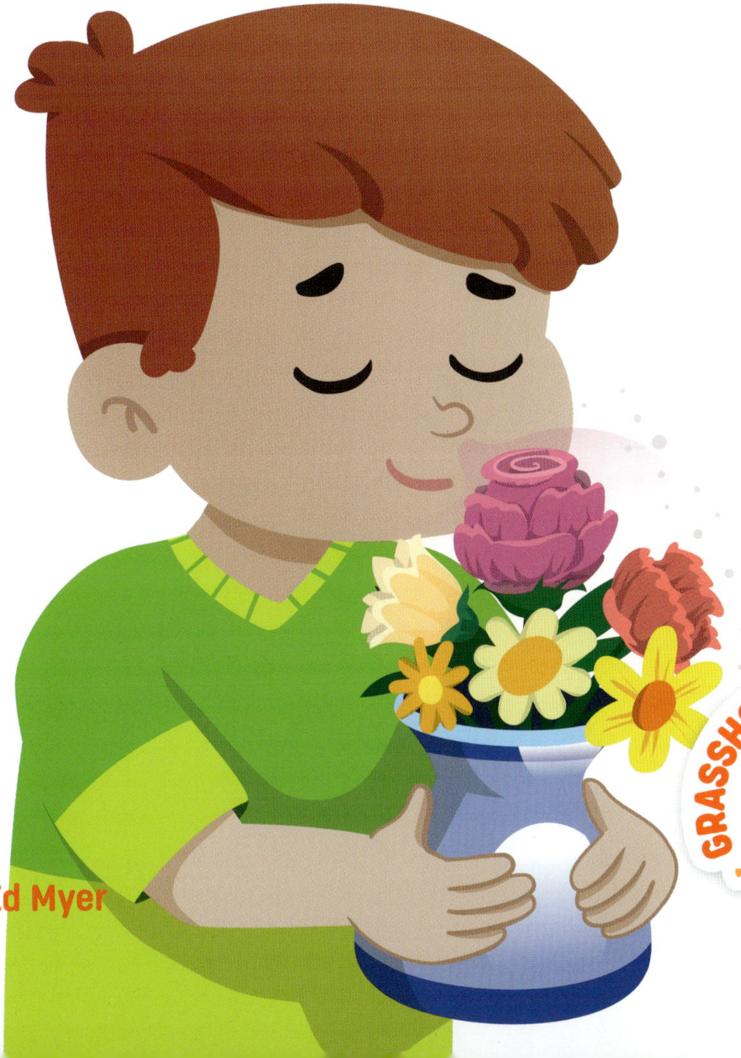

by Mari Schuh
illustrated by Ed Myer

GRASSHOPPER

Tools for Parents & Teachers

Grasshopper Books enhance imagination and introduce the earliest readers to fiction with fun storylines and illustrations. The easy-to-read text supports early reading experiences with repetitive sentence patterns and sight words.

Before Reading
- Discuss the cover illustration. What do they see?
- Look at the glossary together. Discuss the words.

Read the Book
- Read the book to the child, or have him or her read independently.
- "Walk" through the book and look at the illustrations. Who is the main character? What is happening in the story?

After Reading
- Prompt the child to think more. Ask: Think about all the things you do in a day. What did your nervous system tell your body to do today?

Grasshopper Books are published by Jump!
5357 Penn Avenue South
Minneapolis, MN 55419
www.jumplibrary.com

Copyright © 2022 Jump! International copyright reserved in all countries. No part of this book may be reproduced in any form without written permission from the publisher.

Library of Congress Cataloging-in-Publication Data

Names: Schuh, Mari C., 1975- author.
Myer, Ed, illustrator.
Title: Noah's nifty nervous system / by Mari Schuh; illustrated by Ed Myer.
Description: Minneapolis, MN: Jump!, Inc., [2022]
Series: Let's look at body systems!
Includes index.
Audience: Ages 7-10
Identifiers: LCCN 2021038015 (print)
LCCN 2021038016 (ebook)
ISBN 9781636906478 (hardcover)
ISBN 9781636906485 (paperback)
ISBN 9781636906492 (ebook)
Subjects: LCSH: Nervous system–Juvenile literature.
Brain–Juvenile literature.
Classification: LCC QP361.5 .S38 2022 (print)
LCC QP361.5 (ebook)
DDC 612.8–dc23
LC record available at https://lccn.loc.gov/2021038015
LC ebook record available at https://lccn.loc.gov/2021038016

Editor: Jenna Gleisner
Direction and Layout: Anna Peterson
Illustrator: Ed Myer

Printed in the United States of America at Corporate Graphics in North Mankato, Minnesota.

Table of Contents

Sending Messages 4

Where in the Body? 22

Let's Review! 23

To Learn More 23

Glossary 24

Index 24

Sending Messages

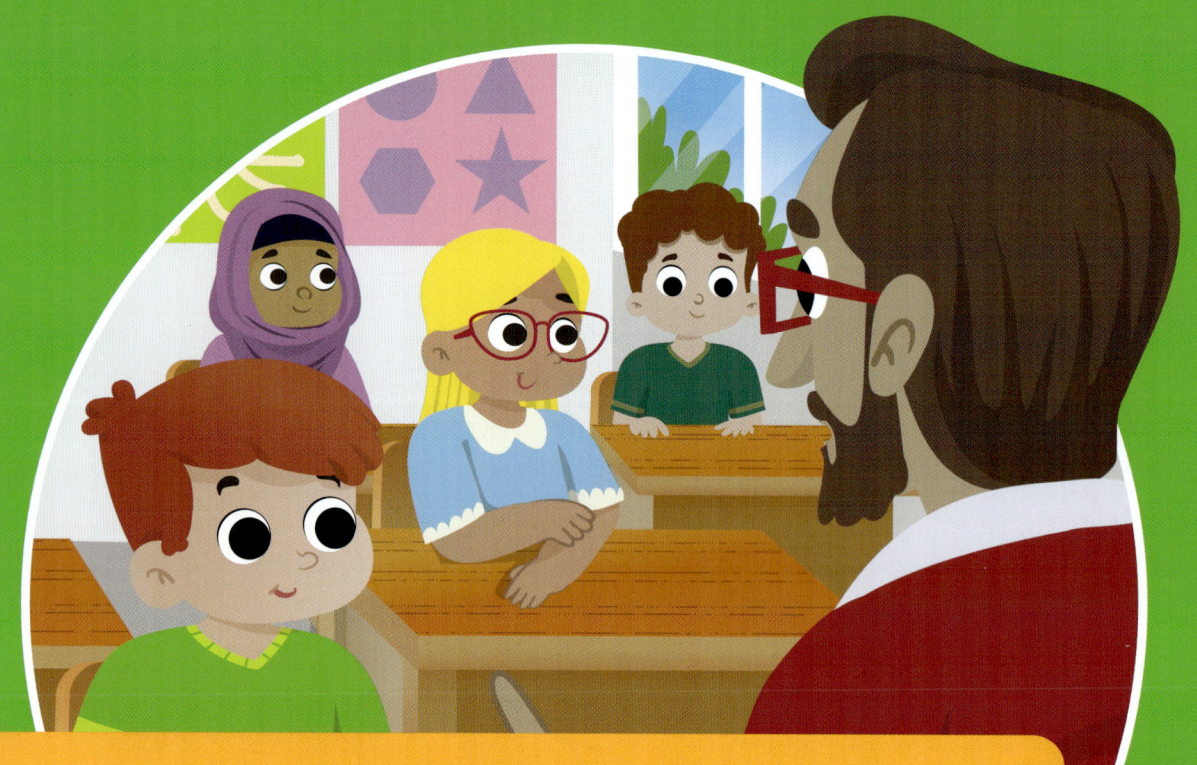

"Hello, class! Today we're going to learn about the nervous system," says Mr. Rajab. "But first, I'd like to know what you did over the weekend."

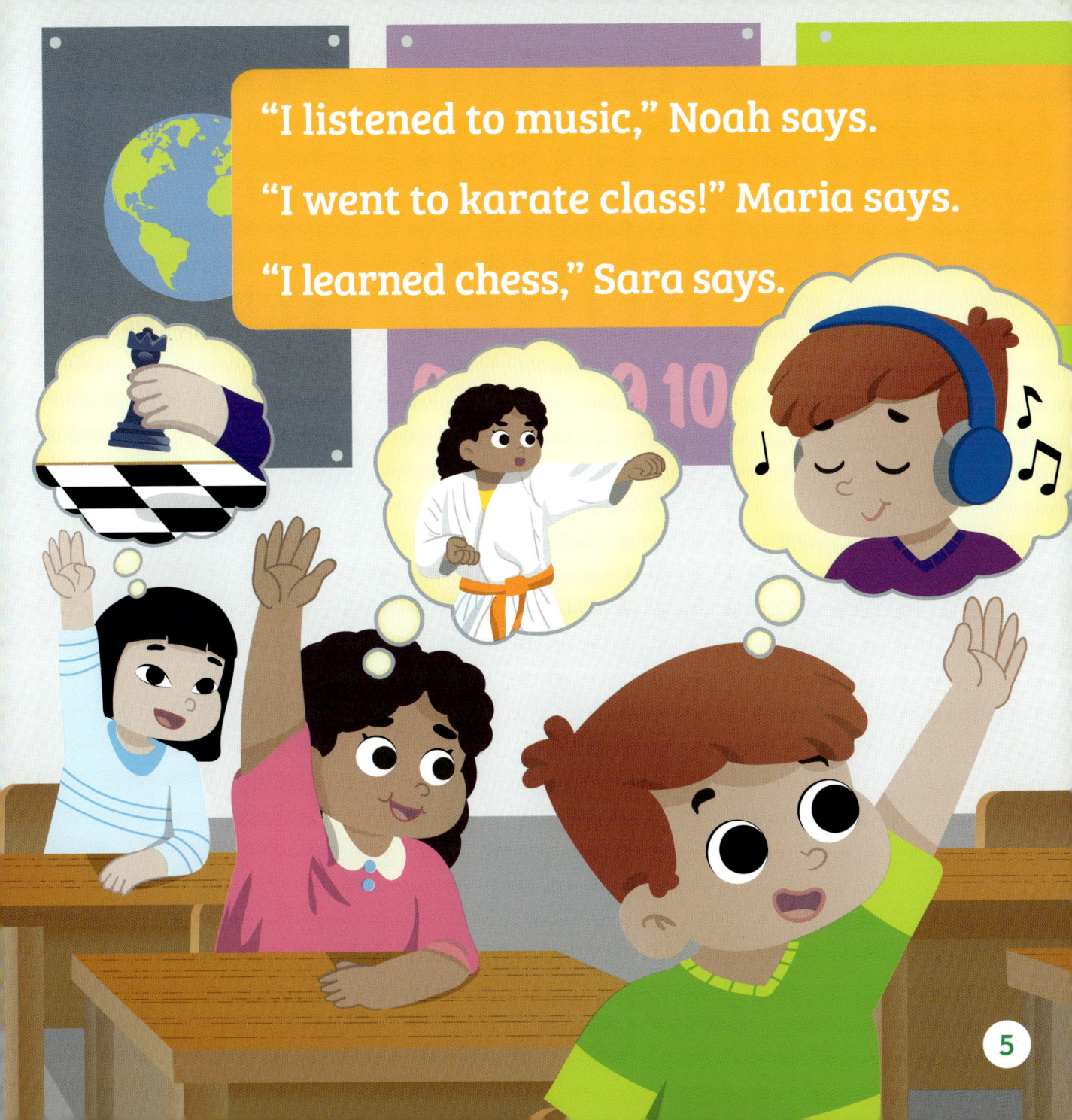

"Did you know that your nervous system helped you do all those things?" Mr. Rajab asks.

"How?" asks Sara.

"It begins with the brain. Your brain is the leader of your nervous system," Mr. Rajab says.

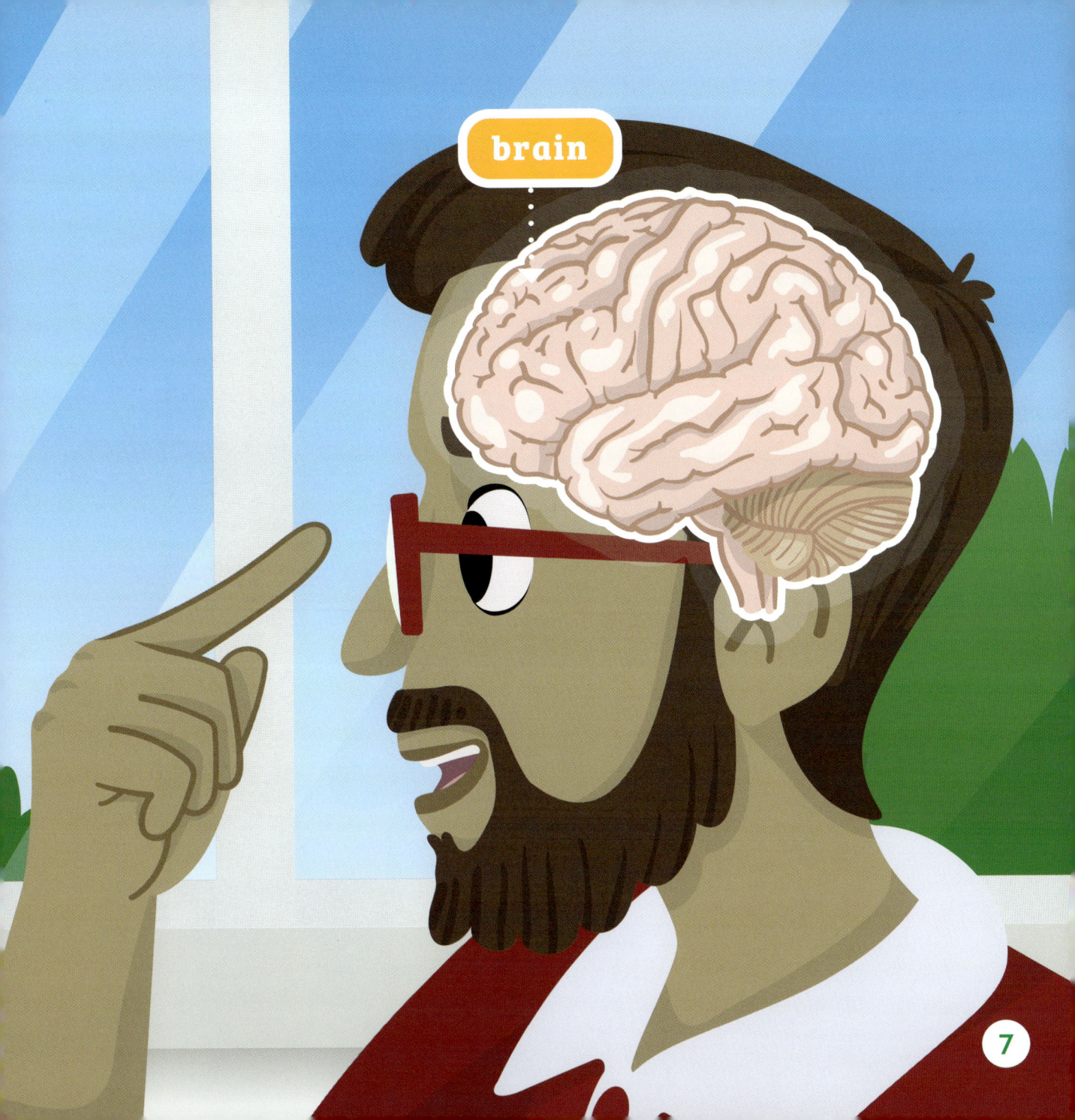

"Your brain connects to your spinal cord. This long, flexible tube links your brain and your body's nerves," he continues.

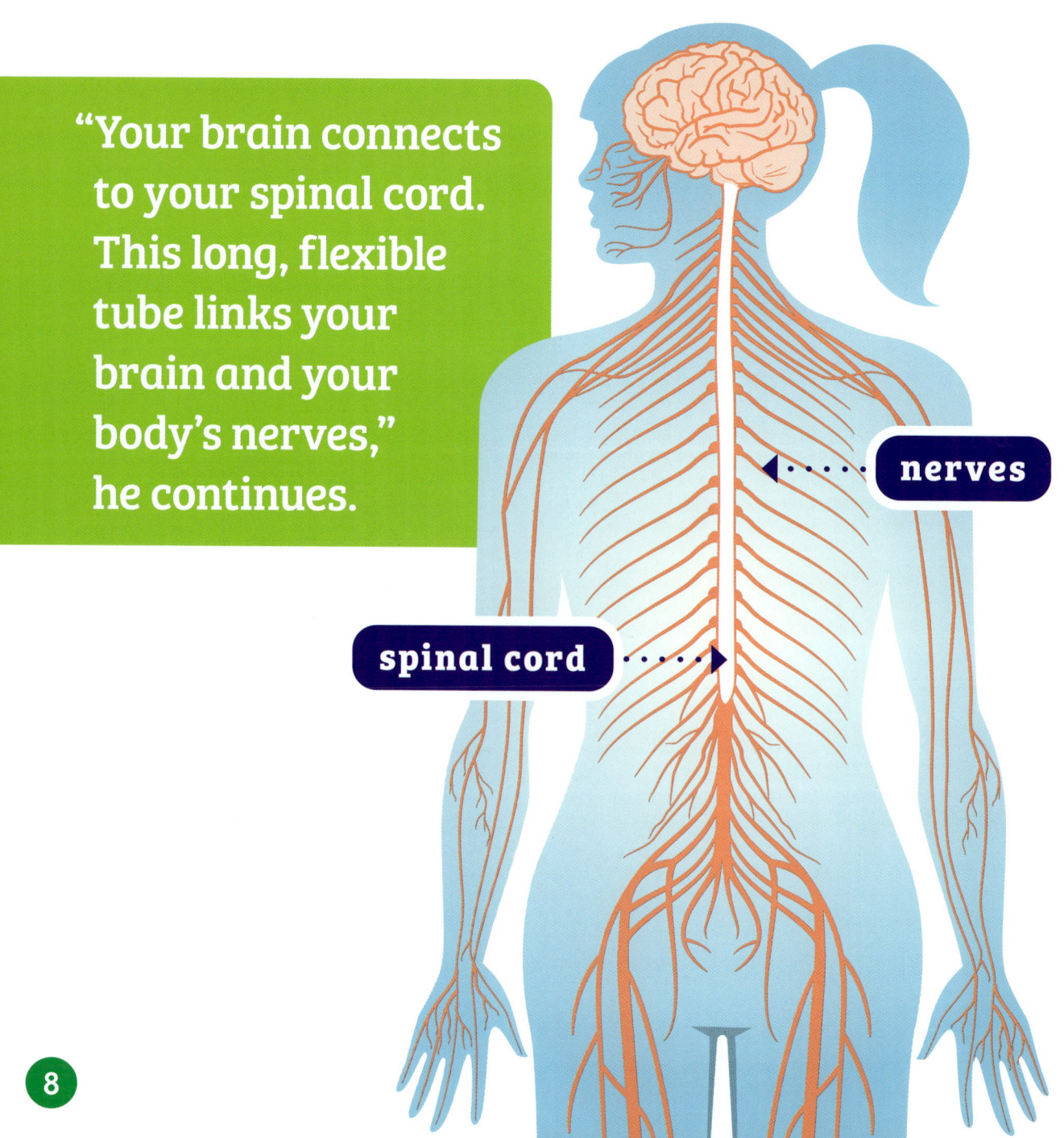

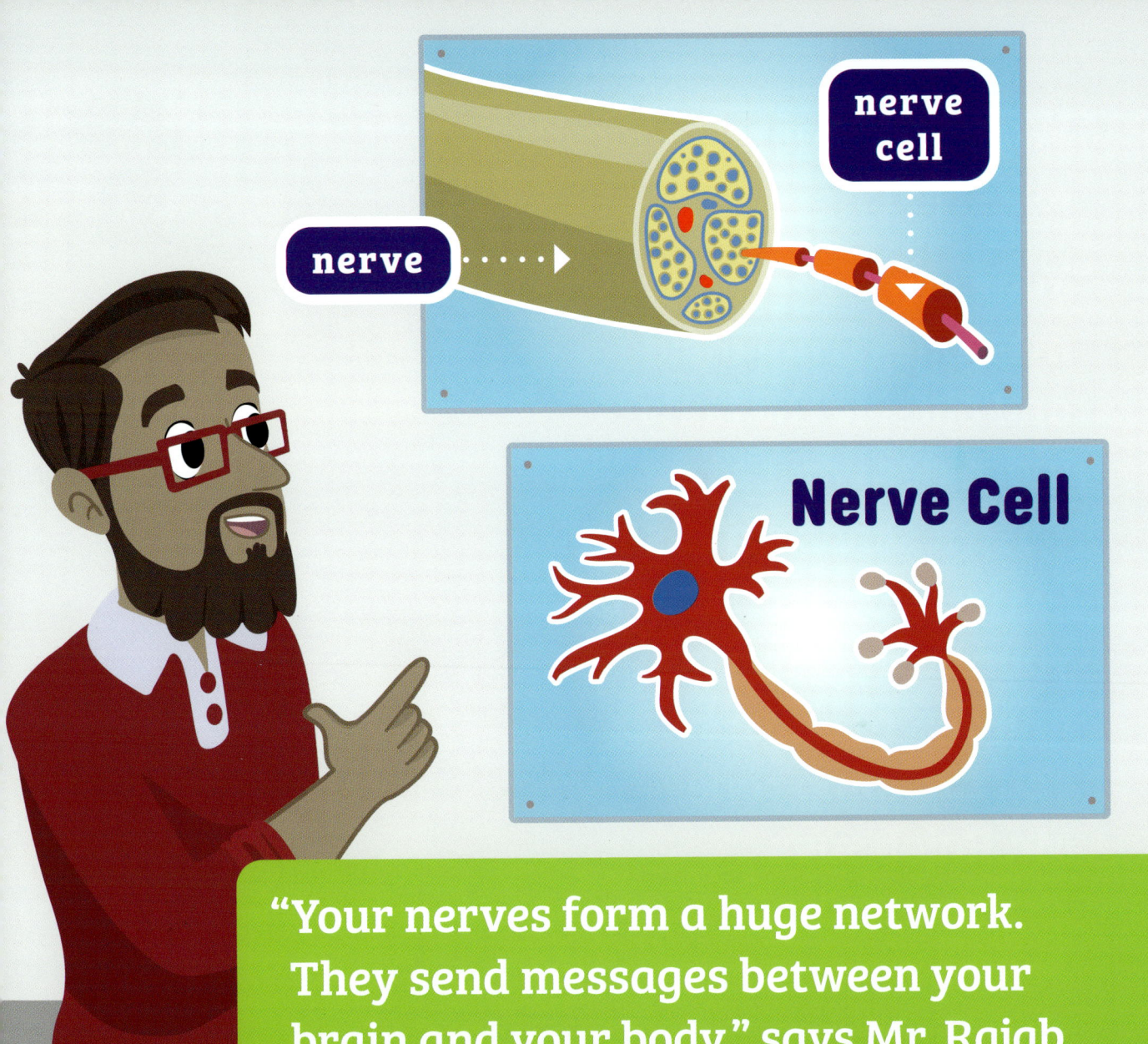

"Your nerves form a huge network. They send messages between your brain and your body," says Mr. Rajab.

"What kinds of messages?" asks Noah.

"Your brain receives messages from inside and outside the body. It decides what to do. Then it sends a message to the body. For example, your brain tells your muscles to move so you can jump rope," Mr. Rajab says.

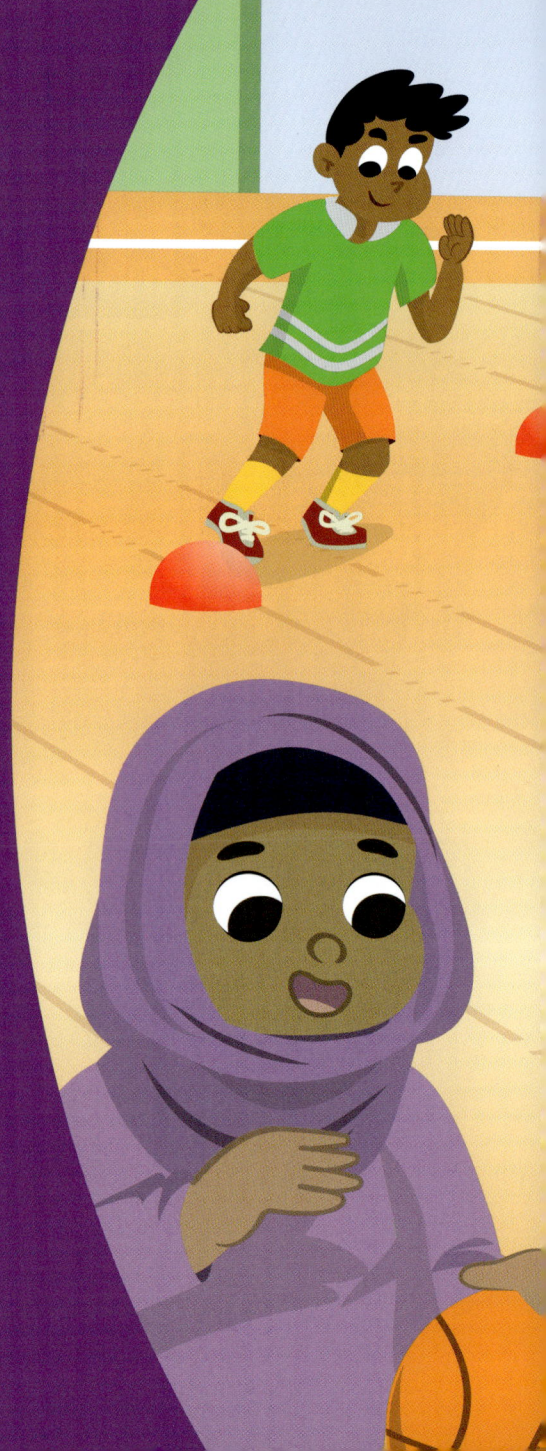

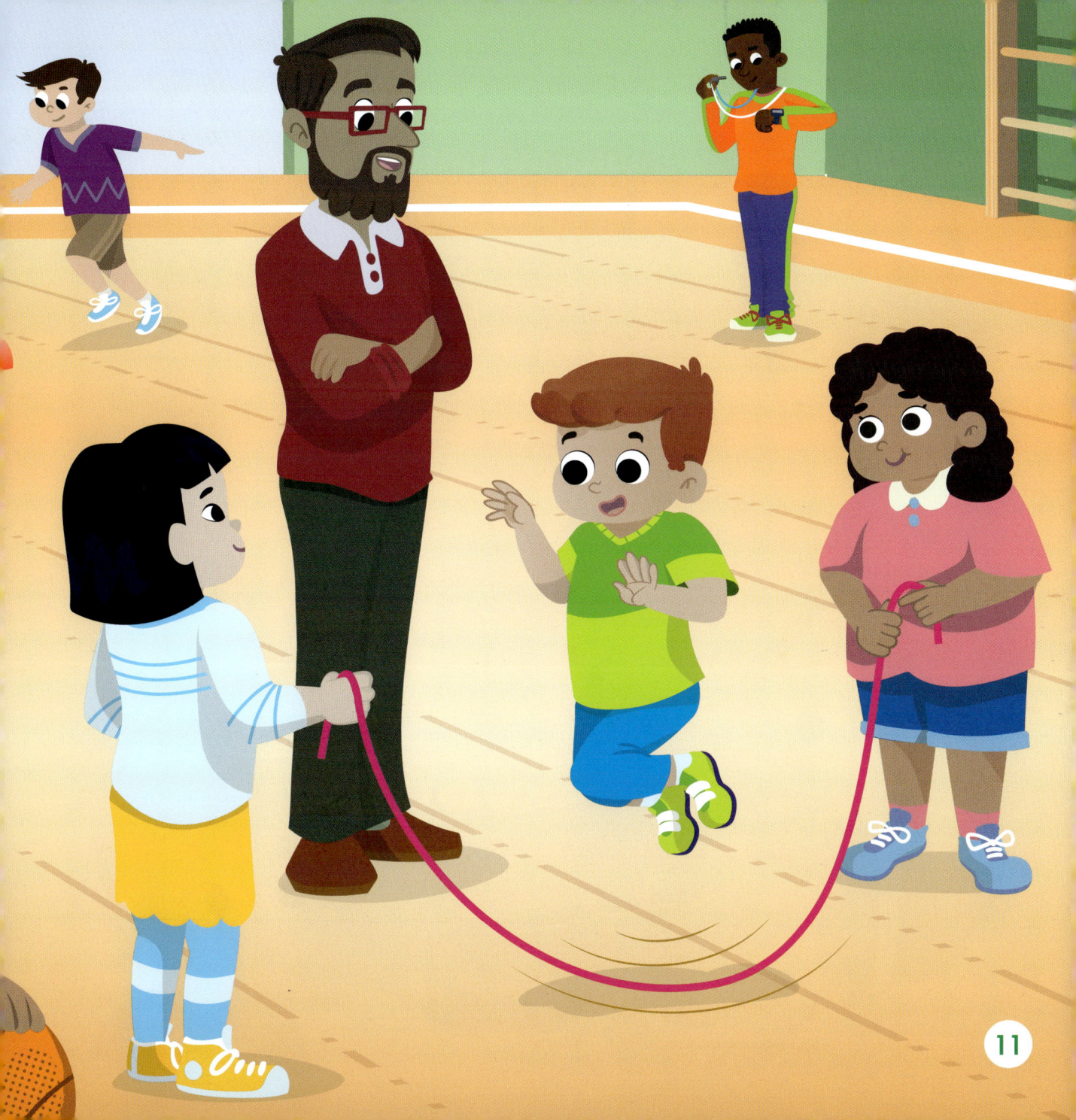

"So I have my nervous system to thank when I almost touch something hot?" asks Noah.

"Yes! Without any thought, nerves in your fingers send messages to your spinal cord," Mr. Rajab says.

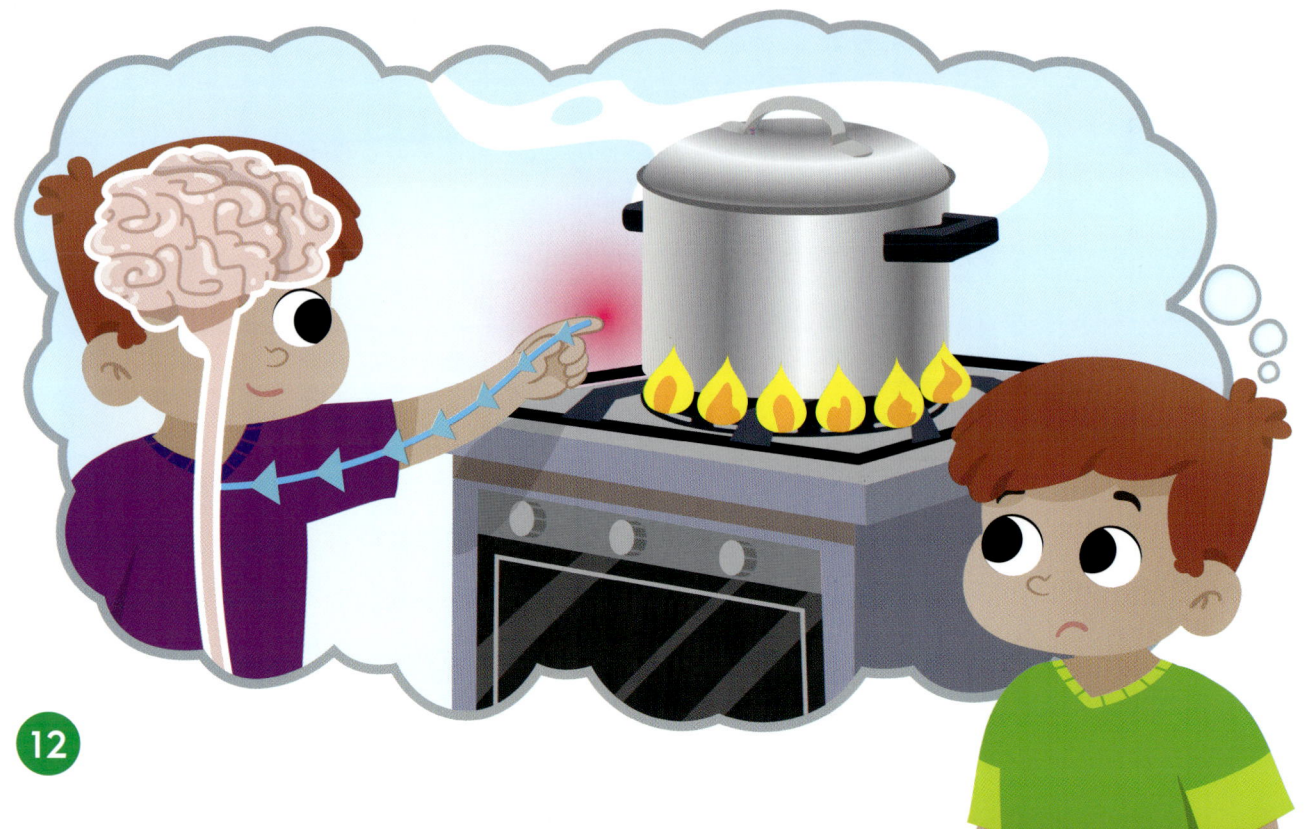

"Then your spinal cord sends messages to your muscles to move your hand. It's called a reflex. It happens very quickly!" Mr. Rajab explains. "This helps keep you safe."

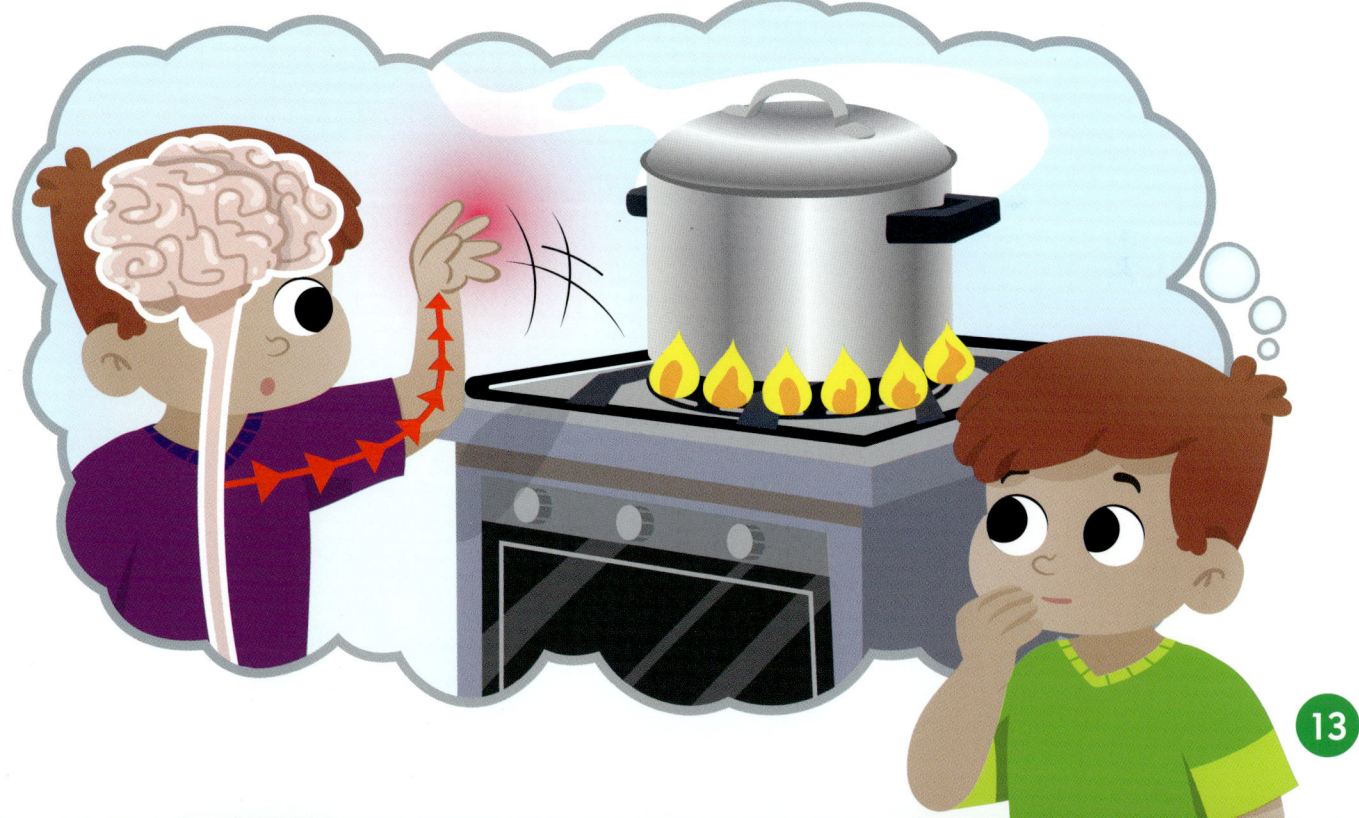

"The nervous system sounds like a control center," says Maria.

"It is!" says Mr. Rajab. "It controls nearly everything you do, think, say, and feel. It even controls your senses. Your eyes, ears, and other body parts send messages to your brain. What do you see, hear, feel, touch, and smell right now?"

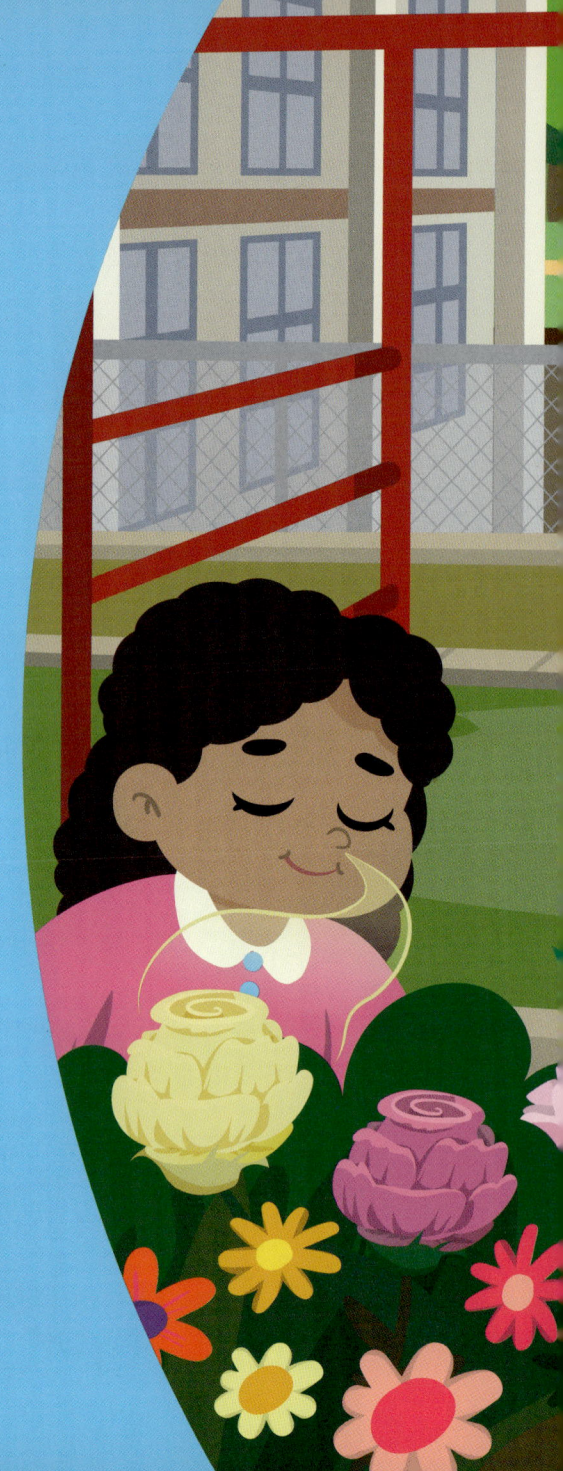

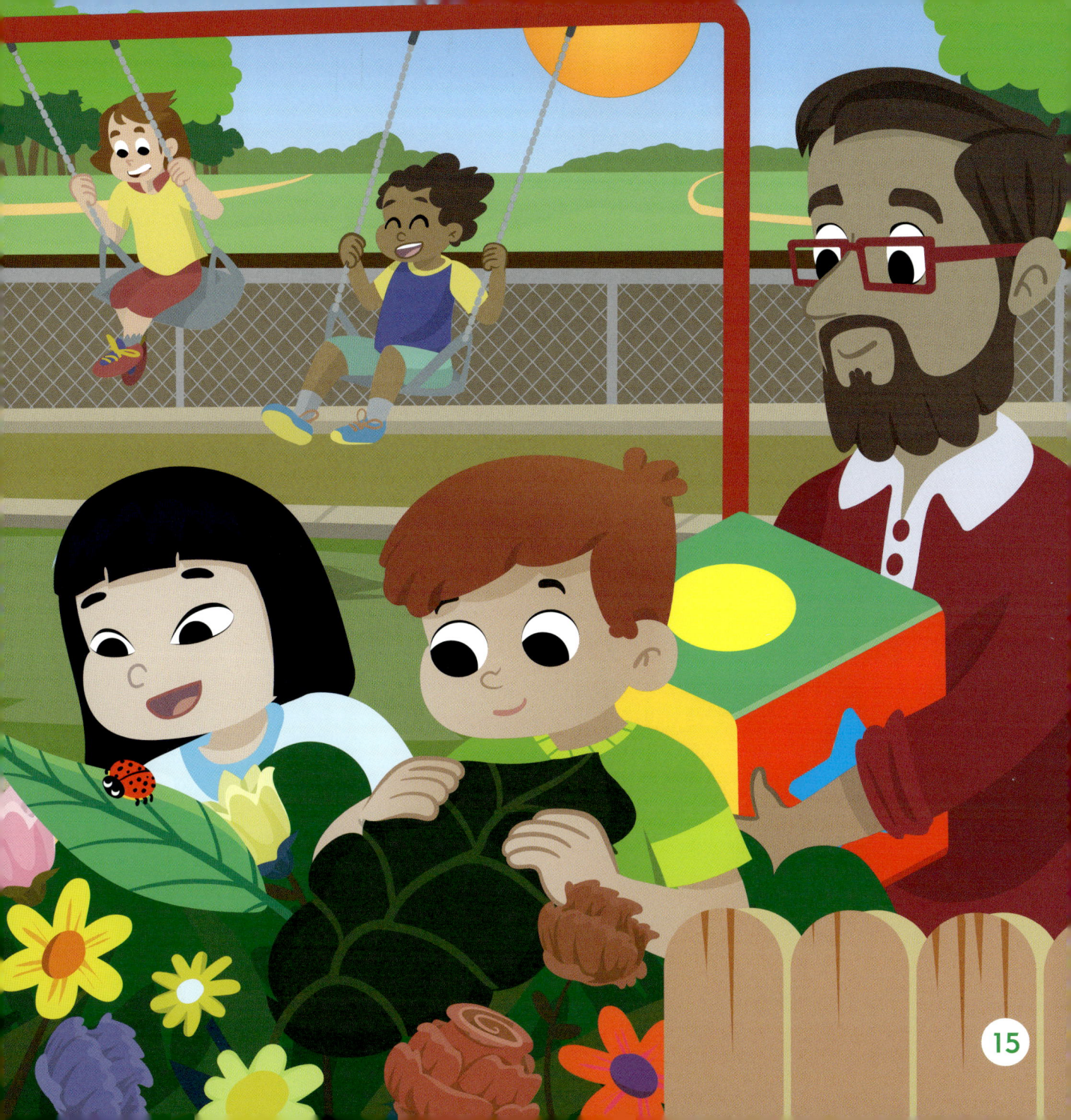

"Does my nervous system ever take a break?" asks Noah.

"It's busy all the time!" Mr. Rajab answers. "Right now, it's helping you learn and remember. Tonight, it will help you sleep. It even helps you do things you don't think about, like breathe. Pretty nifty, right?"

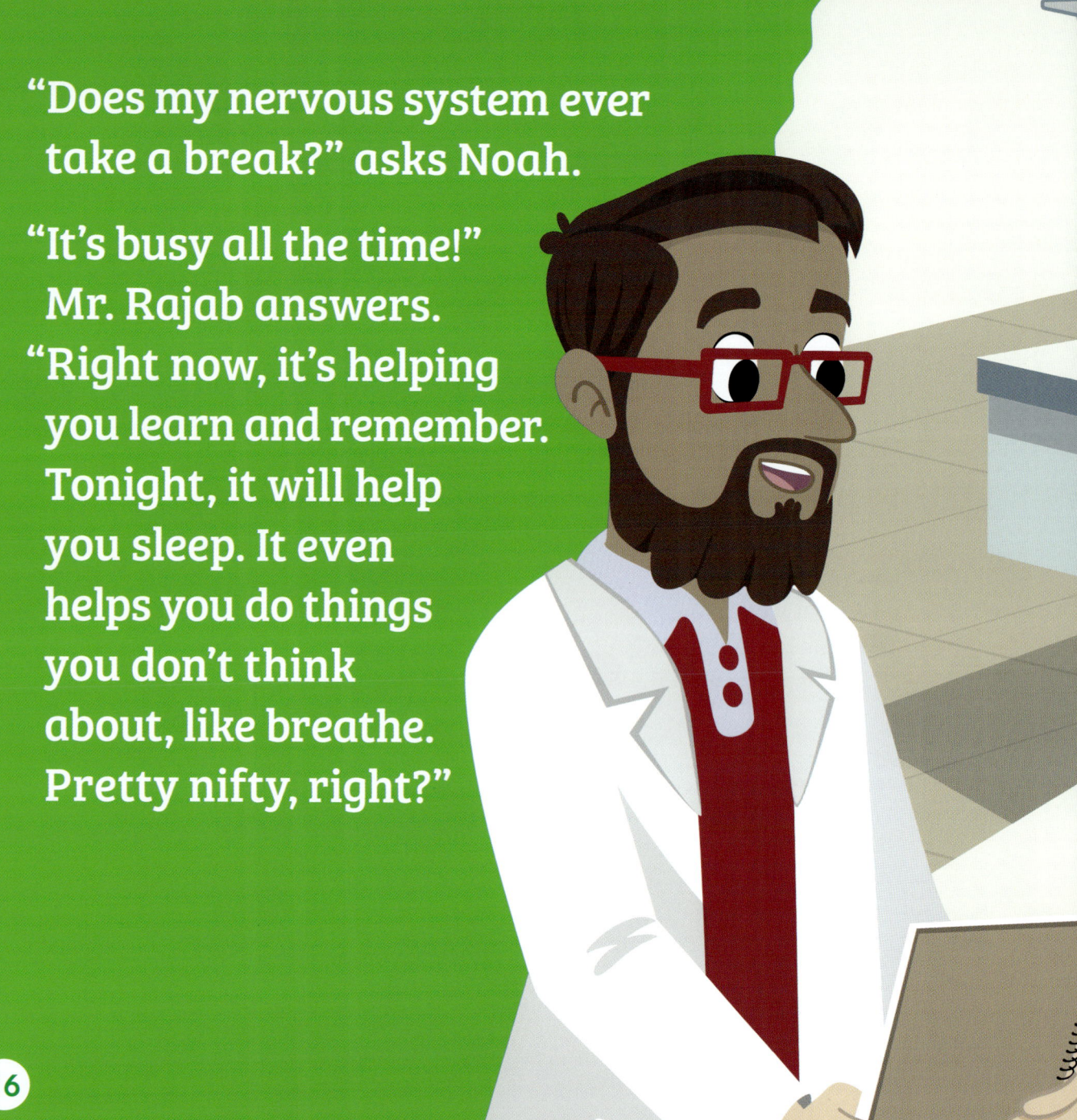

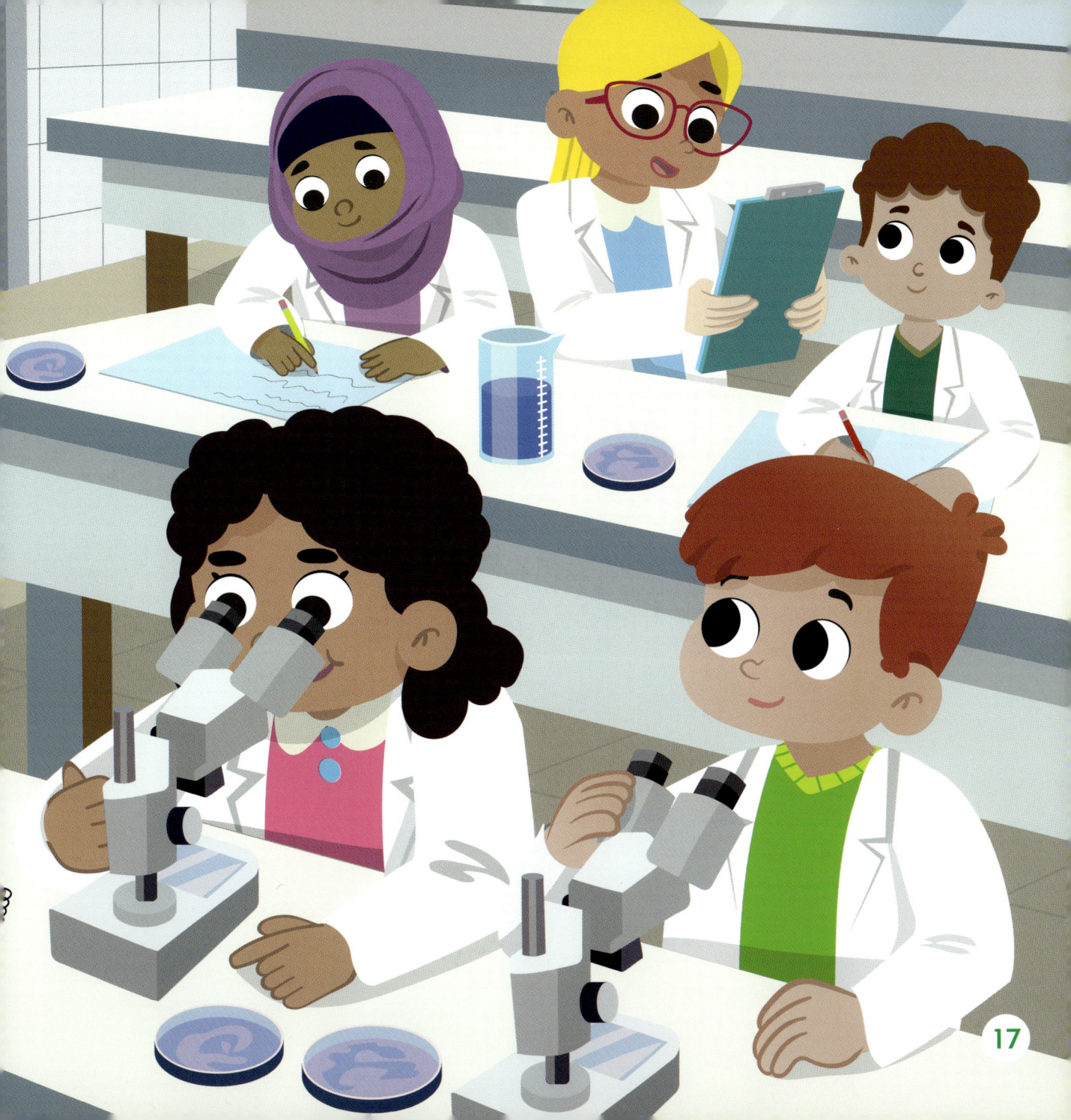

"The nervous system seems super powerful," Maria says.

"It is!" Mr. Rajab says. "It helps you think, learn, talk, and much more. It also lets you remember all sorts of things."

"Like the day I got a puppy!" Maria says.

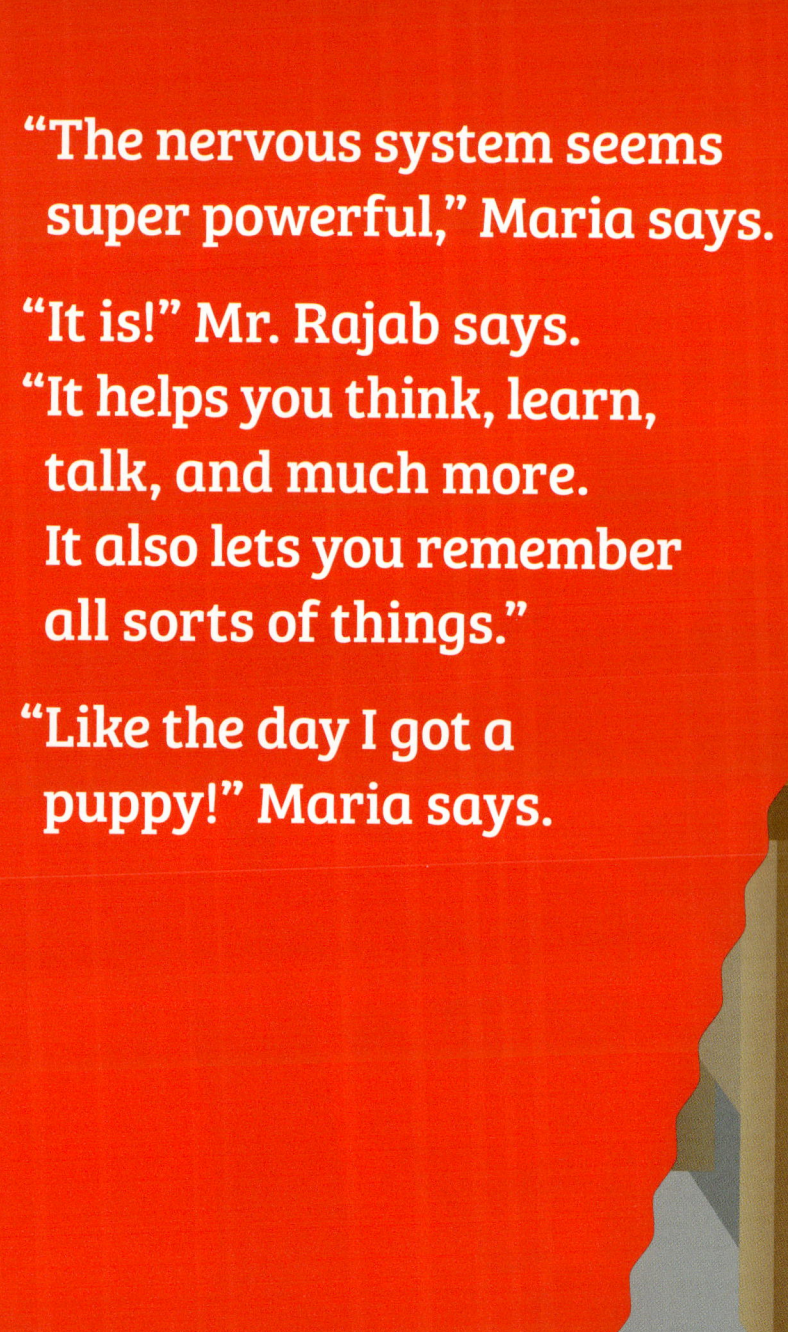

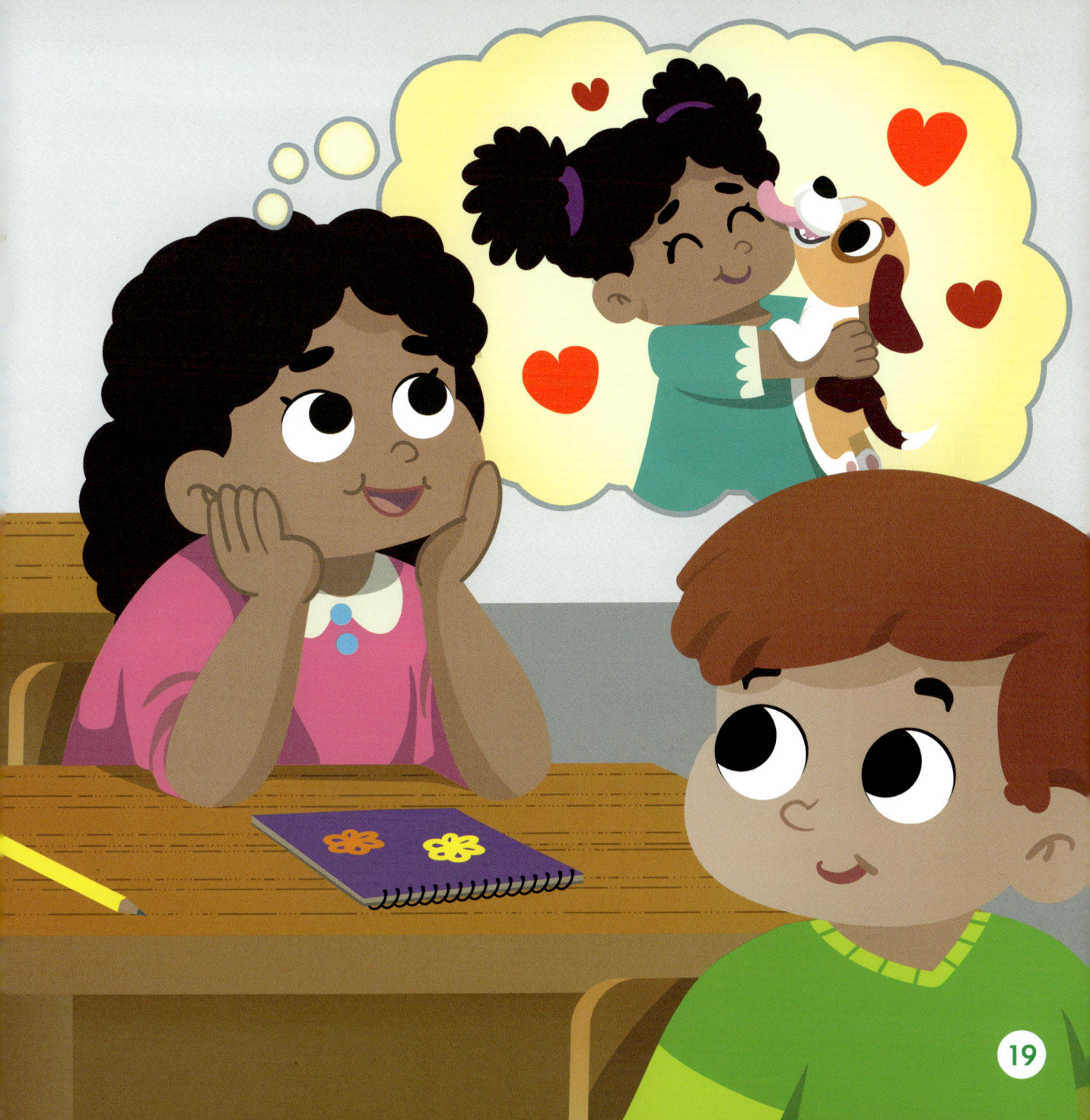

"That's right," Mr. Rajab says. "That's why it's important to take good care of your nervous system. One way is challenging your brain with puzzles. Let's see who can finish their puzzle first!"

"I will!" Noah says. "My nervous system will help me!"

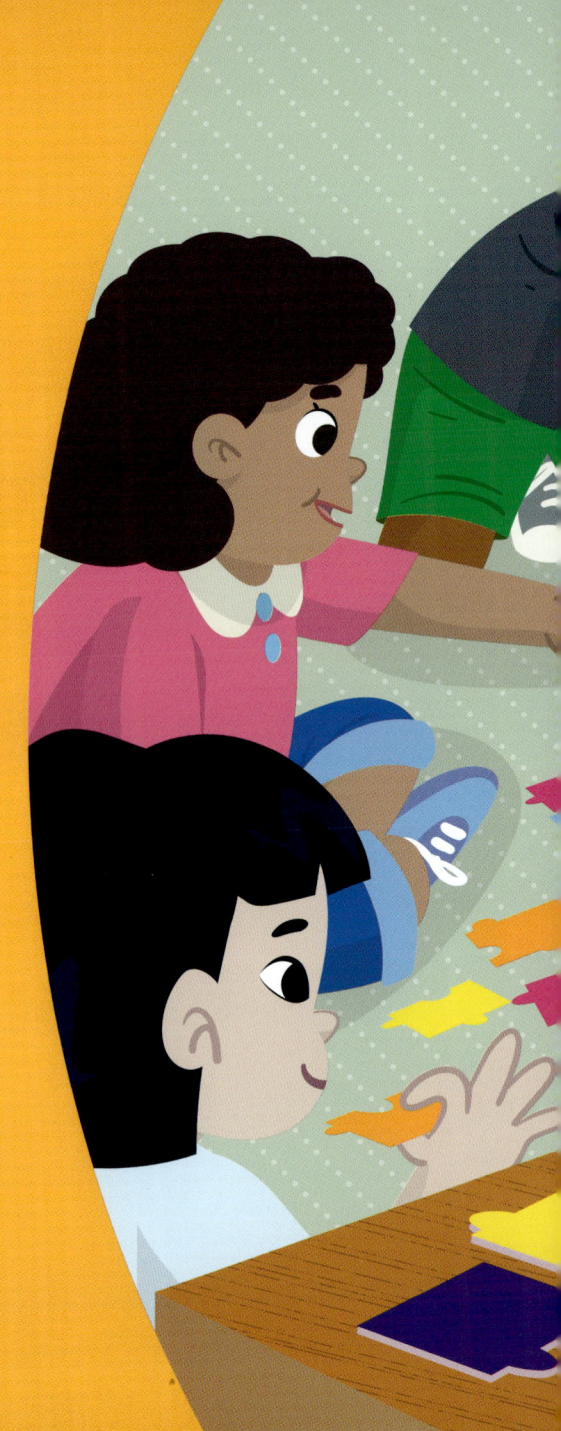

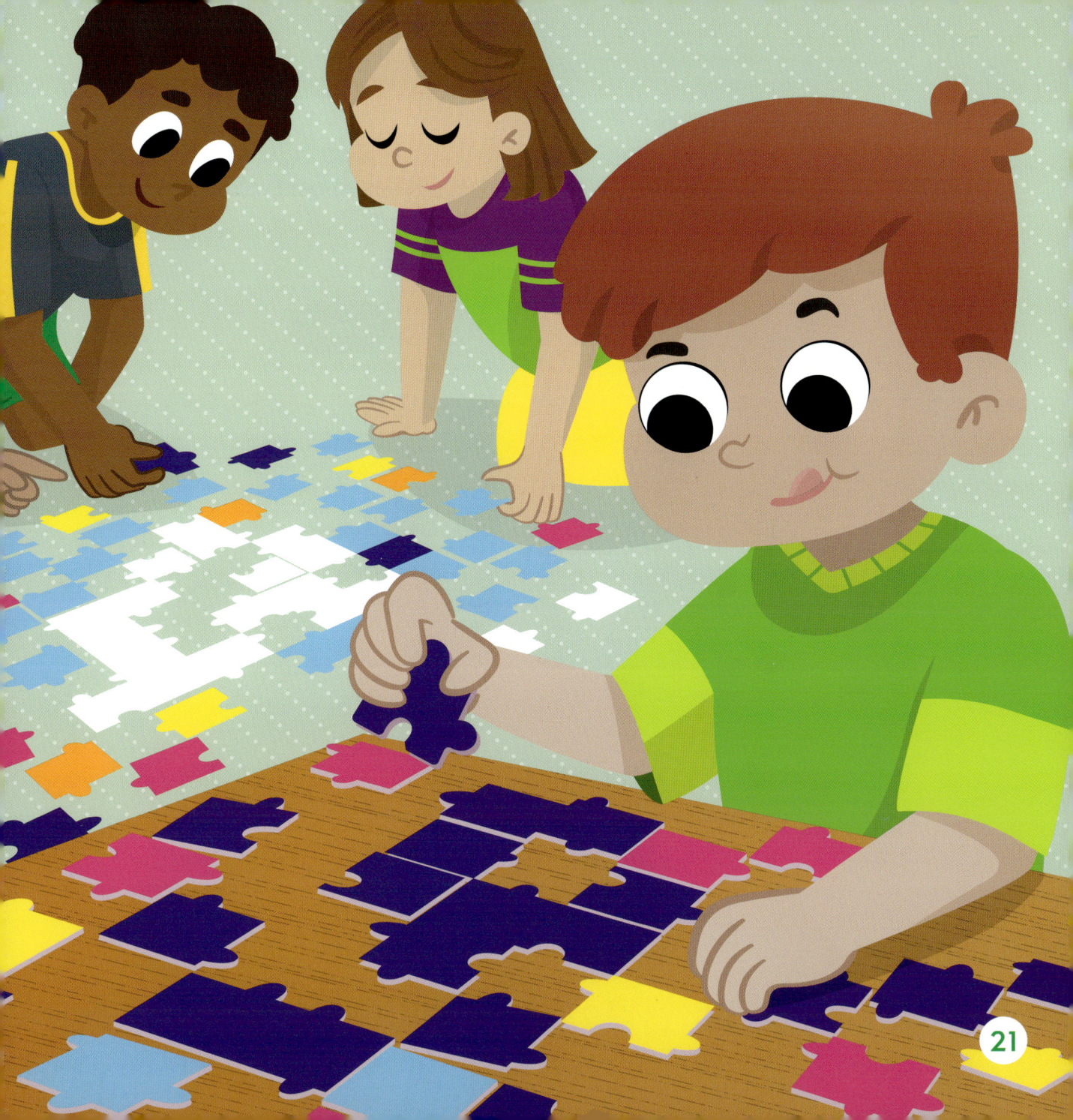

Where in the Body?

Your brain, spinal cord, and nerves work together to control nearly everything your body does. Take a look!

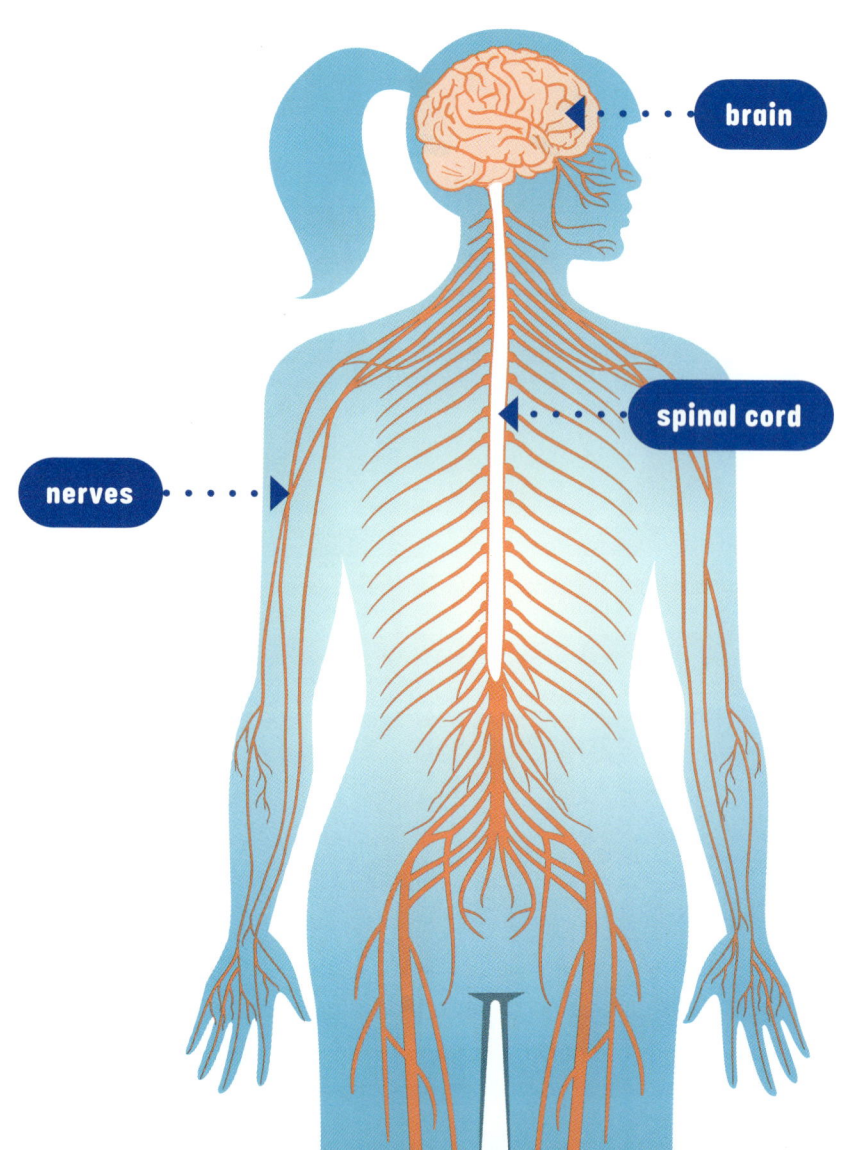

Let's Review!

Below are some of the actions the nervous system helps us do. What other actions does the nervous system help with?

- learning something new 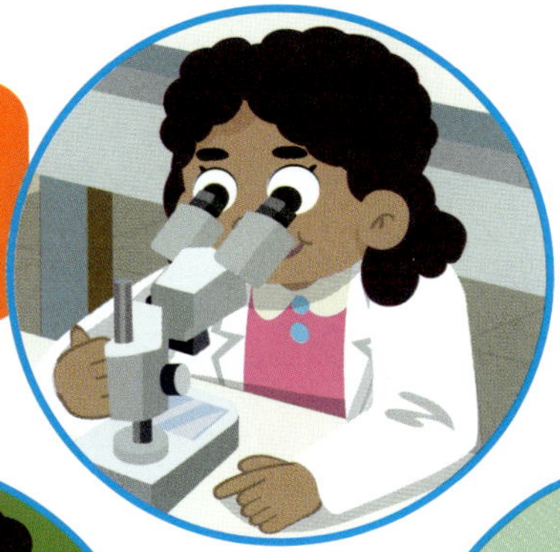
- moving your body 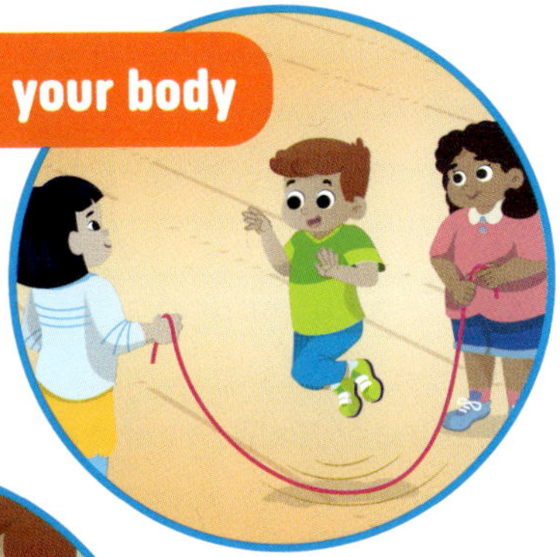 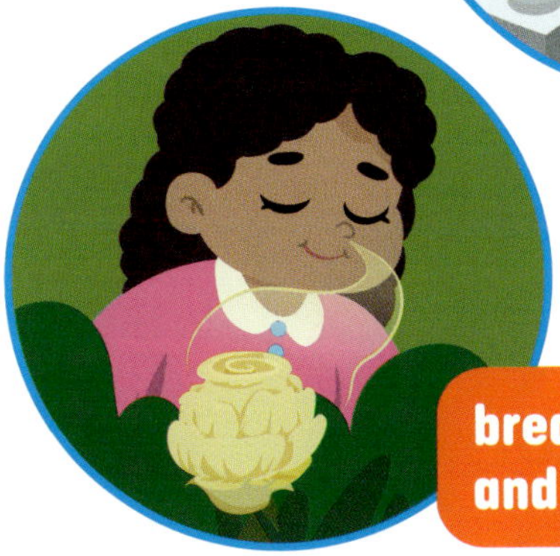
- breathing and smelling 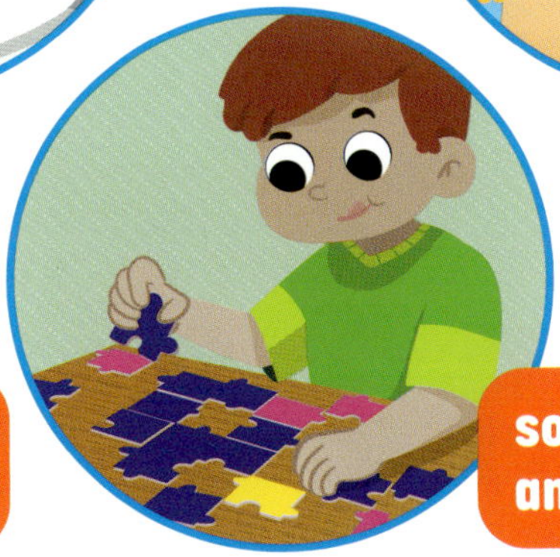
- solving puzzles and problems

To Learn More

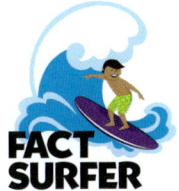

Finding more information is as easy as 1, 2, 3.

1. Go to www.factsurfer.com
2. Enter "**Noah'sniftynervoussystem**" into the search box.
3. Choose your book to see a list of websites.

Glossary

brain: The organ inside your skull that controls your body's activities as well as your thoughts, memories, and emotions.

flexible: Able to bend.

muscles: Tissues in the body that can contract, or shorten and tighten, to produce movement.

nerves: Threads of nerve cells that carry messages between the brain and other parts of your body so you can move and feel.

reflex: An automatic action or movement that happens without a person's control of effort.

spinal cord: A thick cord of nerves that runs down the spine and connects the brain to the body.

Index

body 8, 9, 10, 14
brain 6, 8, 9, 10, 14, 20
breathe 16
feel 14
hear 14
learn 4, 5, 16, 18
listened 5
messages 9, 10, 12, 13, 14
muscles 10, 13
nerves 8, 9, 12

puzzles 20
reflex 13
remember 16, 18
see 14
senses 14
sleep 16
smell 14
spinal cord 8, 12, 13
think 14, 16, 18
touch 12, 14